The Definitive Mediterranean Cookbook to Snacks and Appetizers

Get Ready to Enjoy your Moments of Break with Fast and Delicious Meals

Alia Compton

contained within this document, including, but not limited to, — errors, omissions, or inaccuracies.

Table of contents

Cucumber Sandwich Bites

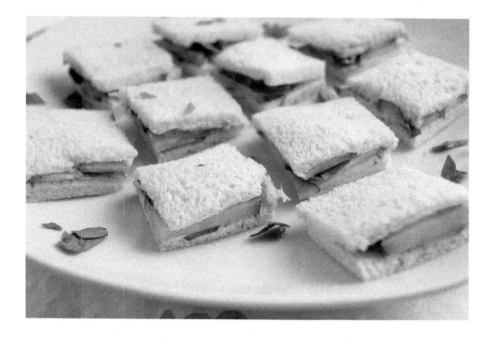

Difficulty Level: 1/5

Preparation time: *5 minutes*

Servings: *12*

Ingredients:

1 cucumber, sliced

8 slices whole wheat bread

2 tablespoons cream cheese, soft

1 tablespoon chives, chopped

¼ cup avocado, peeled, pitted and mashed

1 teaspoon mustard

Salt and black pepper to the taste

Directions:

Spread the mashed avocado on each bread slice, also spread the rest of the ingredients except the cucumber slices.

Divide the cucumber slices on the bread slices, cut each slice in thirds, arrange on a platter and serve as an appetizer.

Nutrition:

Calories: 187

Fat: 12.4g

Fiber: 2.1g

Carbohydrates: 4.5g

Protein: 8.2g

Yogurt Dip

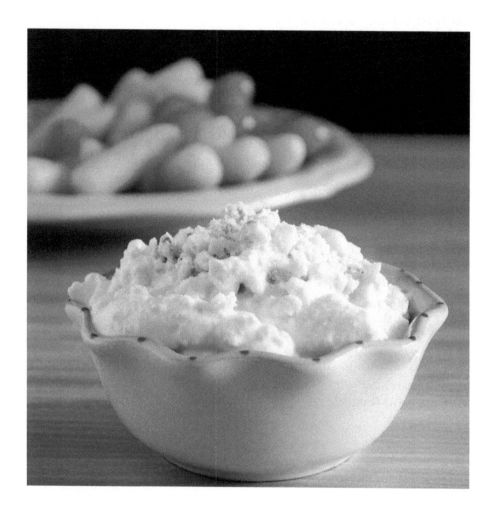

Difficulty Level: 1/5

Preparation time: *10 minutes*

Cooking time: *0 minutes*

Servings: 6

Ingredients:

2 cups Greek yogurt

2 tablespoons pistachios, toasted and chopped

A pinch of salt and white pepper

2 tablespoons mint, chopped

1 tablespoon kalamata olives, pitted and chopped

¼ cup za'atar spice

¼ cup pomegranate seeds

1/3 cup olive oil

Directions:

In a bowl, combine the yogurt with the pistachios and the rest of the ingredients, whisk well, divide into small cups and serve with pita chips on the side.

Nutrition:

Calories: 294

Fat: 18g

Fiber: 1g

Carbohydrates: 2g

Protein: 10g

Tomato Bruschetta

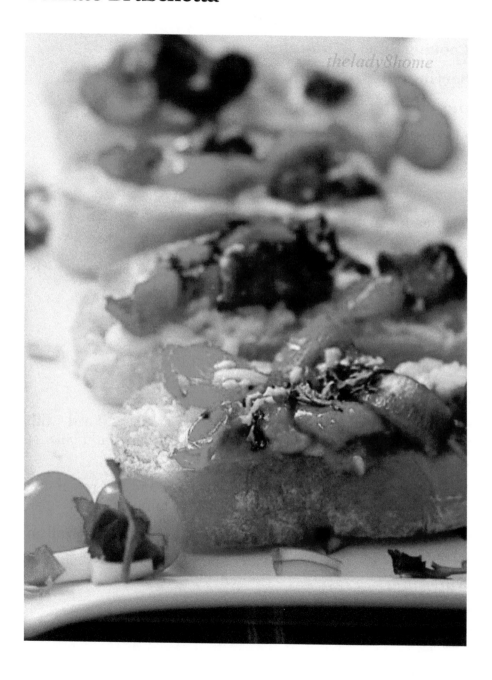

Difficulty Level: 2/5

Preparation time: *10 minutes*

Cooking time: *10 minutes*

Servings: *6*

Ingredients:

1 baguette, sliced

1/3 cup basil, chopped

6 tomatoes, cubed

2 garlic cloves, minced

A pinch of salt and black pepper

1 teaspoon olive oil

1 tablespoon balsamic vinegar

½ teaspoon garlic powder

Cooking spray

Directions:

Arrange the baguette slices on a baking sheet lined with parchment paper, grease them with cooking spray and bake at 400 degrees F for 10 minutes.

In a bowl, mix the tomatoes with the basil and the remaining ingredients, toss well and leave aside for 10 minutes.

Divide the tomato mix on each baguette slice, arrange them all on a platter and serve.

Nutrition:

Calories: 162

Fat: 4g

Fiber: 7g

Carbohydrates: 29g

Protein: 4g

Olives and Cheese Stuffed Tomatoes

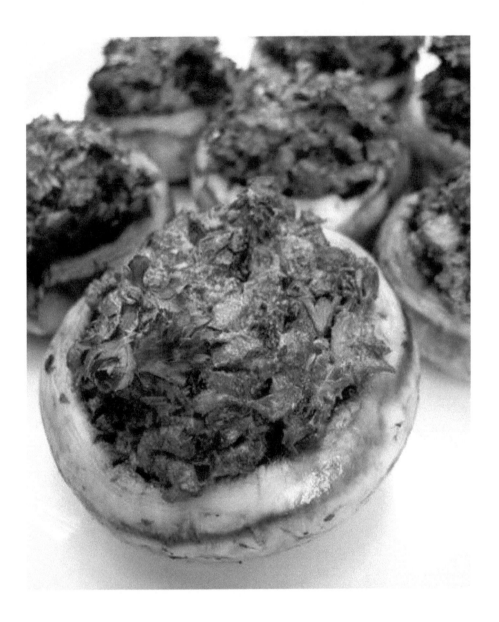

Difficulty Level: 1/5

Preparation time: *10 minutes*

Servings: 24

Ingredients:

24 cherry tomatoes, top cut off and insides scooped out

2 tablespoons olive oil

¼ teaspoon red pepper flakes

½ cup feta cheese, crumbled

2 tablespoons black olive paste

¼ cup mint, torn

Directions:

In a bowl, mix the olives paste with the rest of the ingredients except the cherry tomatoes and whisk well.

Stuff the cherry tomatoes with this mix, arrange them all on a platter and serve as an appetizer.

Nutrition:

Calories 136

Fat: 8.6g

Fiber: 4.8g

Carbohydrates: 5.6g

Protein: 5.1g

Red Pepper Tapenade

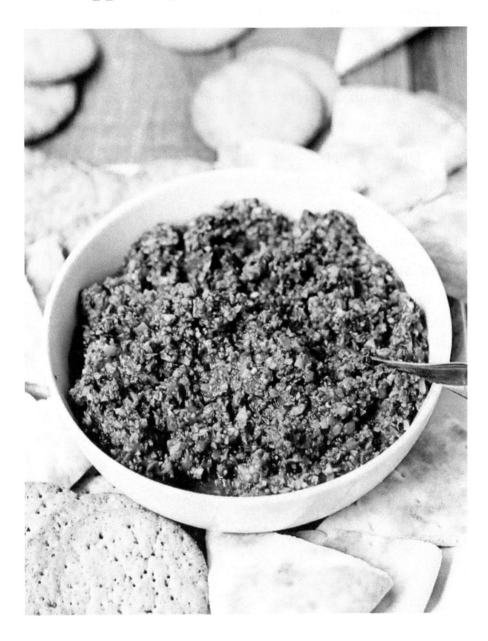

Difficulty Level: 1/5

Preparation time: *10 minutes*

Cooking time: *0 minutes*

Servings: *4*

Ingredients:

7 ounces roasted red peppers, chopped

½ cup parmesan, grated

1/3 cup parsley, chopped

14 ounces canned artichokes, drained and chopped

3 tablespoons olive oil

¼ cup capers, drained

1 and ½ tablespoons lemon juice

2 garlic cloves, minced

Directions:

In your blender, combine the red peppers with the parmesan and the rest of the ingredients and pulse well.

Divide into cups and serve as a snack.

Nutrition:

Calories: 200

Fat: 5.6g

Fiber: 4.5g

Carbohydrates: 12.4g

Protein: 4.6g

Coriander Falafel

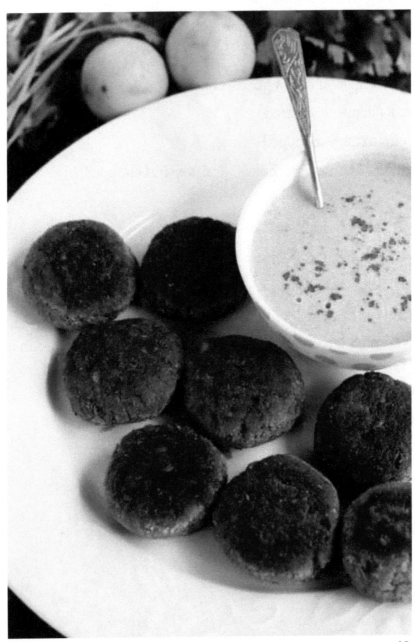

Difficulty Level: 2/5

Preparation time: *10 minutes*

Cooking time: *10 minutes*

Servings: *8*

Ingredients:

1 cup canned garbanzo beans, drained and rinsed

1 bunch parsley leaves

1 yellow onion, chopped

5 garlic cloves, minced

1 teaspoon coriander, ground

A pinch of salt and black pepper

¼ teaspoon cayenne pepper

¼ teaspoon baking soda

¼ teaspoon cumin powder

1 teaspoon lemon juice

3 tablespoons tapioca flour

Olive oil for frying

Directions:

In your food processor, combine the beans with the parsley, onion and the rest the ingredients except the oil and the flour and pulse well.

Transfer the mix to a bowl, add the flour, stir well, shape 16 balls out of this mix and flatten them a bit.

Heat up a pan with some oil over medium-high heat, add the falafels, cook them for 5 minutes on each side, transfer to paper towels, drain excess grease, arrange them on a platter and serve as an appetizer.

Nutrition:

Calories: 112

Fat: 6.2g

Fiber: 2g

Carbohydrates: 12.3g

Protein: 3.1g

Red Pepper Hummus

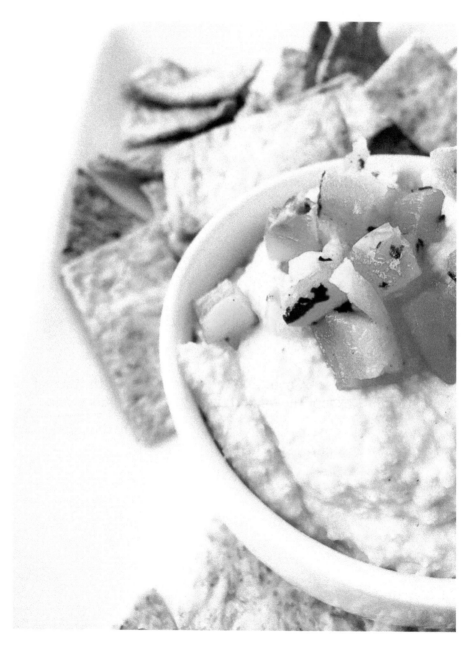

Difficulty Level: 1/5

Preparation time: *10 minutes*

Cooking time: *0 minutes*

Servings: 6

Ingredients:

6 ounces roasted red peppers, peeled and chopped

16 ounces canned chickpeas, drained and rinsed

¼ cup Greek yogurt

3 tablespoons tahini paste

Juice of 1 lemon

3 garlic cloves, minced

1 tablespoon olive oil

A pinch of salt and black pepper

1 tablespoon parsley, chopped

Directions:

In your food processor, combine the red peppers with the rest of the ingredients except the oil and the parsley and pulse well.

Add the oil, pulse again, divide into cups, sprinkle the parsley on top and serve as a party spread.

Nutrition:

Calories: 255

Fat: 11.4g

Fiber: 4.5g

Carbohydrates: 17.4g

Protein: 6.5g

White Bean Dip

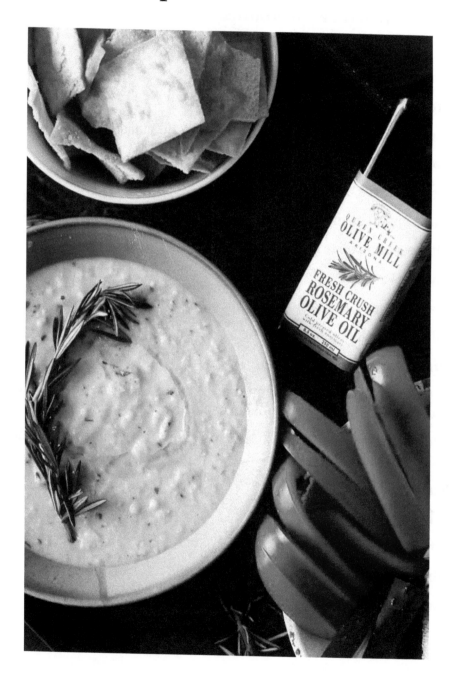

Difficulty Level: 1/5

Preparation time: *10 minutes*

Cooking time: *0 minutes*

Servings: *4*

Ingredients:

15 ounces canned white beans, drained and rinsed

6 ounces canned artichoke hearts, drained and quartered

4 garlic cloves, minced

1 tablespoon basil, chopped

2 tablespoons olive oil

Juice of ½ lemon

Zest of ½ lemon, grated

Salt and black pepper to the taste

Directions:

In your food processor, combine the beans with the artichokes and the rest of the ingredients except the oil and pulse well.

Add the oil gradually, pulse the mix again, divide into cups and serve as a party dip.

Nutrition:

Calories 27

Fat: 11.7g

Fiber: 6.5g

Carbohydrates: 18.5g

Protein: 16.5g

Hummus with Ground Lamb

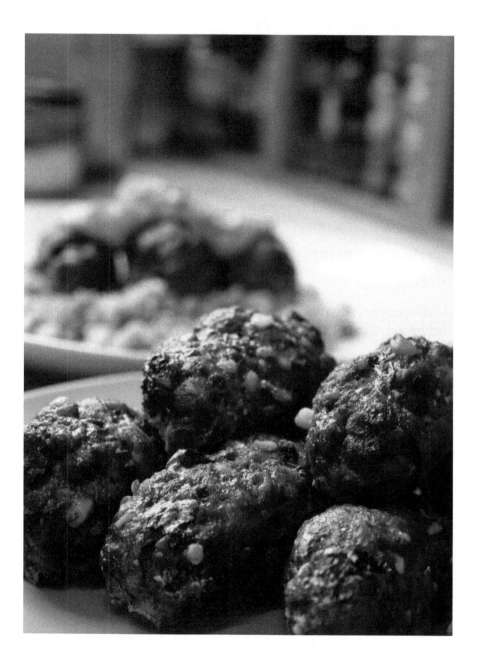

Difficulty Level: 2/5

Preparation time: *10 minutes*

Cooking time: *15 minutes*

Servings: *8*

Ingredients:

10 ounces hummus

12 ounces lamb meat, ground

½ cup pomegranate seeds

¼ cup parsley, chopped

1 tablespoon olive oil

Pita chips for serving

Directions:

Heat up a pan with the oil over medium-high heat, add the meat, and brown for 15 minutes stirring often.

Spread the hummus on a platter, spread the ground lamb all over, also spread the pomegranate seeds and the parsley and serve with pita chips as a snack.

Nutrition:

Calories 133

Fat: 9.7g

Fiber: 1.7g

Carbohydrates: 6.4g

Protein: 5.4g

Eggplant Dip

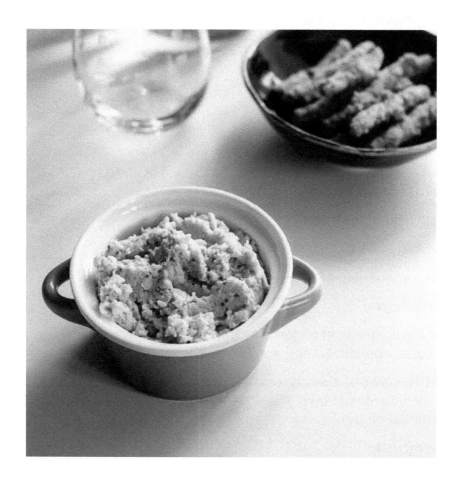

Difficulty Level: 2/5

Preparation time: *10 minutes*

Cooking time: *40 minutes*

Servings: *4*

Ingredients:

1 eggplant, poked with a fork

2 tablespoons tahini paste

2 tablespoons lemon juice

2 garlic cloves, minced

1 tablespoon olive oil

Salt and black pepper to the taste

1 tablespoon parsley, chopped

Directions:

Put the eggplant in a roasting pan, bake at 400 degrees F for 40 minutes, cool down, peel and transfer to your food processor.

Add the rest of the ingredients except the parsley, pulse well, divide into small bowls and serve as an appetizer with the parsley sprinkled on top.

Nutrition:

Calories: 121

Fat: 4.3g

Fiber: 1g

Carbohydrates: 1.4g

Protein: 4.3g

Veggie Fritters

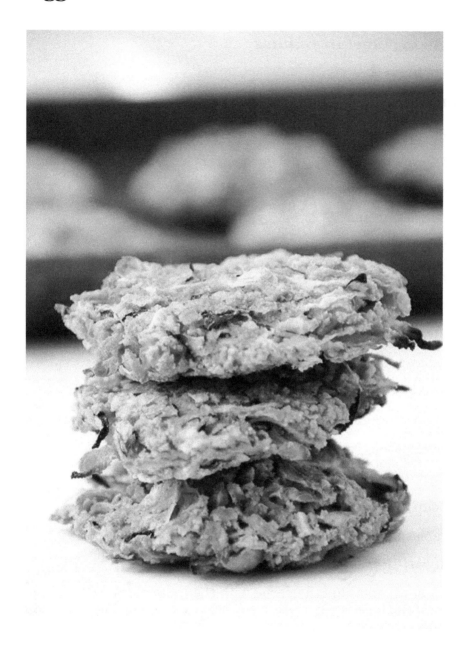

Difficulty Level: 2/5

Preparation time: *10 minutes*

Cooking time: *10 minutes*

Servings: *8*

Ingredients:

2 garlic cloves, minced

2 yellow onions, chopped

4 scallions, chopped

2 carrots, grated

2 teaspoons cumin, ground

½ teaspoon turmeric powder

Salt and black pepper to the taste

¼ teaspoon coriander, ground

2 tablespoons parsley, chopped

¼ teaspoon lemon juice

½ cup almond flour

2 beets, peeled and grated

2 eggs, whisked

¼ cup tapioca flour

3 tablespoons olive oil

Directions:

In a bowl, combine the garlic with the onions, scallions and the rest of the ingredients except the oil, stir well and shape medium fritters out of this mix.

Heat up a pan with the oil over medium-high heat, add the fritters, cook for 5 minutes on each side, arrange on a platter and serve.

Nutrition:

Calories: 209

Fat: 11.2g

Fiber: 3g

Carbohydrates: 4.4g

Protein: 4.8g

Bulgur Lamb Meatballs

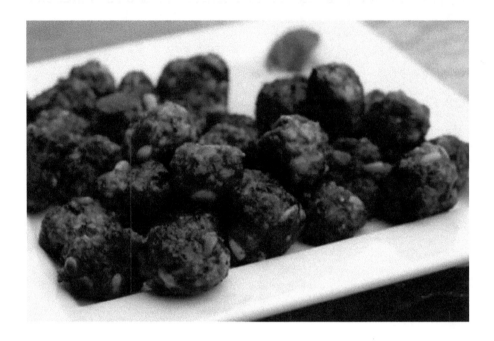

Difficulty Level: 2/5

Preparation time: *10 minutes*

Cooking time: *15 minutes*

Servings: 6

Ingredients:

1 and ½ cups Greek yogurt

½ teaspoon cumin, ground

1 cup cucumber, shredded

½ teaspoon garlic, minced

A pinch of salt and black pepper

1 cup bulgur

2 cups water

1 pound lamb, ground

¼ cup parsley, chopped

¼ cup shallots, chopped

½ teaspoon allspice, ground

½ teaspoon cinnamon powder

1 tablespoon olive oil

Directions:

In a bowl, combine the bulgur with the water, cover the bowl, leave aside for 10 minutes, drain and transfer to a bowl.

Add the meat, the yogurt and the rest of the ingredients except the oil, stir well and shape medium meatballs out of this mix.

Heat up a pan with the oil over medium-high heat, add the meatballs, cook them for 7 minutes on each side, arrange them all on a platter and serve as an appetizer.

Nutrition:

Calories: 300

Fat: 9.6g

Fiber: 4.6g

Carbohydrates: 22.6g

Protein: 6.6g

Cucumber Bites

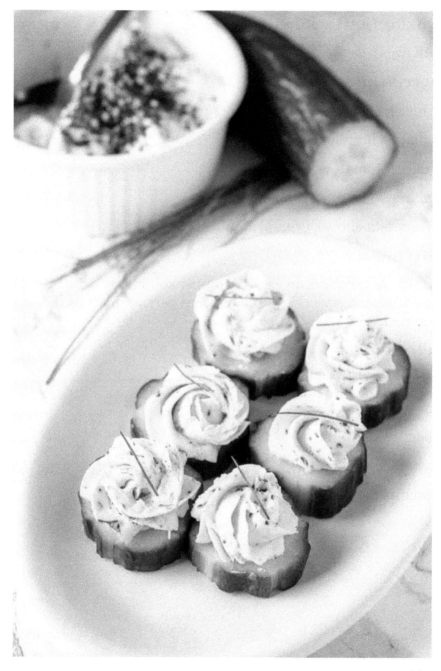

Difficulty Level: 1/5

Preparation time: *10 minutes*

Cooking time: *0 minutes*

Servings: *12*

Ingredients:

1 English cucumber, sliced into 32 rounds

10 ounces hummus

16 cherry tomatoes, halved

1 tablespoon parsley, chopped

1 ounce feta cheese, crumbled

Directions:

Spread the hummus on each cucumber round, divide the tomato halves on each, sprinkle the cheese and parsley on to and serve as an appetizer.

Nutrition:

Calories: 162

Fat: 3.4g

Fiber: 2g

Carbohydrates: 6.4g

Protein: 2.4g

Stuffed Avocado

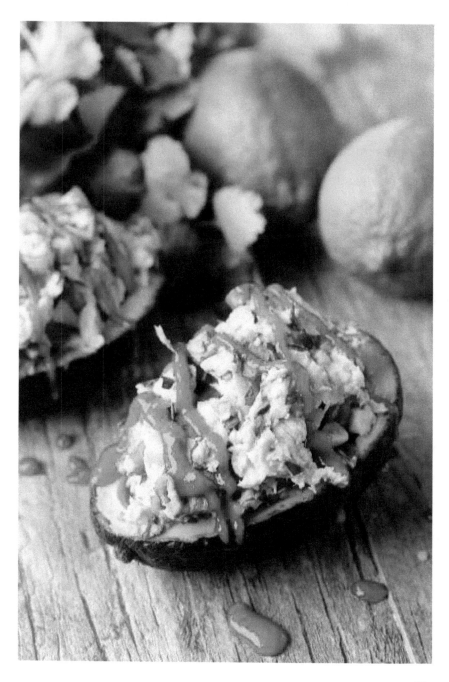

Difficulty Level: 1/5

Preparation time: *10 minutes*

Cooking time: *0 minutes*

Servings: 2

Ingredients:

1 avocado, halved and pitted

10 ounces canned tuna, drained

2 tablespoons sun-dried tomatoes, chopped

1 and ½ tablespoon basil pesto

2 tablespoons black olives, pitted and chopped

Salt and black pepper to the taste

2 teaspoons pine nuts, toasted and chopped

1 tablespoon basil, chopped

Directions:

In a bowl, combine the tuna with the sun-dried tomatoes and the rest of the ingredients except the avocado and stir.

Stuff the avocado halves with the tuna mix and serve as an appetizer.

Nutrition:

Calories: 233

Fat: 9g

Fiber: 3.5g

Carbohydrates: 11.4g

Protein: 5.6g

Wrapped Plums

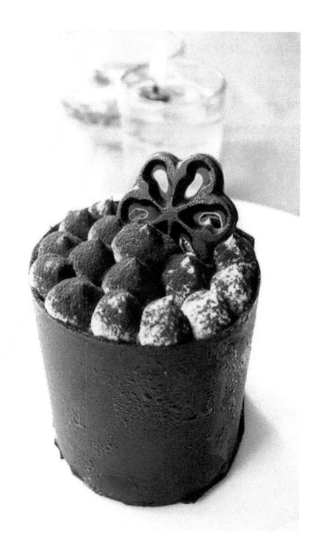

Difficulty Level: 1/5

Preparation time: *5 minutes*

Cooking time: *0 minutes*

Servings: *8*

Ingredients:

2 ounces prosciutto, cut into 16 pieces

4 plums, quartered

1 tablespoon chives, chopped

A pinch of red pepper flakes, crushed

Directions:

Wrap each plum quarter in a prosciutto slice, arrange them all on a platter, sprinkle the chives and pepper flakes all over and serve.

Nutrition:

Calories: 30

Fat: 1g

Fiber: 0g

Carbohydrates: 4g

Protein: 2g

Summer Squash Ribbons with Lemon and Ricotta

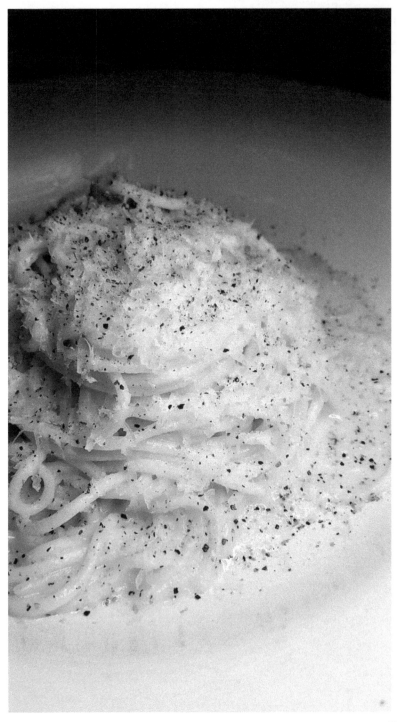

Difficulty Level: 1/5

Preparation time: *20 minutes*

Cooking time: *0 minutes*

Servings: *4*

Ingredients:

2 medium zucchini or yellow squash

½ cup ricotta cheese

2 tablespoons fresh mint, chopped, plus additional mint leaves for garnish

2 tablespoons fresh parsley, chopped

Zest of ½ lemon

2 teaspoons lemon juice

½ teaspoon kosher salt

¼ teaspoon freshly ground black pepper

1 tablespoon extra-virgin olive oil

Directions:

Using a vegetable peeler, make ribbons by peeling the summer squash lengthwise. The squash ribbons will resemble the wide pasta, pappardelle.

In a medium bowl, combine the ricotta cheese, mint, parsley, lemon zest, lemon juice, salt, and black pepper.

Place mounds of the squash ribbons evenly on 4 plates then dollop the ricotta mixture on top. Drizzle with the olive oil and garnish with the mint leaves.

Nutrition:

Calories: 90

Total fat: 6g

Saturated fat: 2g

Cholesterol: 10mg

Sodium: 180mg

Potassium: 315mg

Total Carbohydrates: 5g

Fiber: 1g

Sugars: 3g

Protein: 5g

Magnesium: 25mg

Calcium: 105mg

Sautéed Kale with Tomato and Garlic

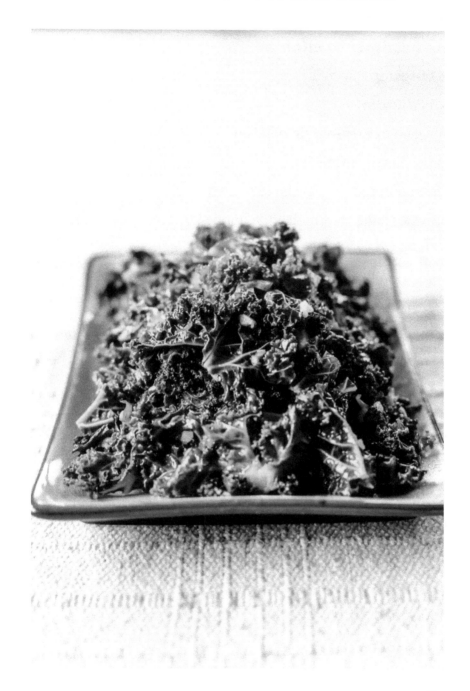

Difficulty Level: 2/5

Preparation time: *5 minutes*

Cooking time: *10 minutes*

Servings: *4*

Ingredients:

1 tablespoon extra-virgin olive oil

4 garlic cloves, sliced

¼ teaspoon red pepper flakes

2 bunches kale, stemmed and chopped or torn into pieces

1 (14.5-ounce) can no-salt-added diced tomatoes

½ teaspoon kosher salt

Directions:

Heat the olive oil in a wok or large skillet over medium-high heat. Add the garlic and red pepper flakes, and sauté until fragrant, about 30 seconds. Add the kale and sauté, about 3 to 5 minutes, until the kale shrinks down a bit.

Add the tomatoes and the salt, stir together, and cook for 3 to 5 minutes, or until the liquid reduces and the kale cooks down further and becomes tender.

INGREDIENT TIP: Adding garlic and red pepper flakes to the oil first allows the flavors to permeate the oil, creating more flavor for the overall dish. If this makes the dish too spicy for your palate, eliminate the red pepper flakes or add them in step 2 with the salt and tomatoes.

Nutrition:

Calories: 110

Total fat: 5g

Saturated fat: 1g

Cholesterol: 0mg

Sodium: 222mg

Potassium: 535mg

Total Carbohydrates: 15g

Fiber: 6g

Sugars: 6g

Protein: 6g

Magnesium: 50mg

Calcium: 182mg

Green Beans with Pine Nuts and Garlic

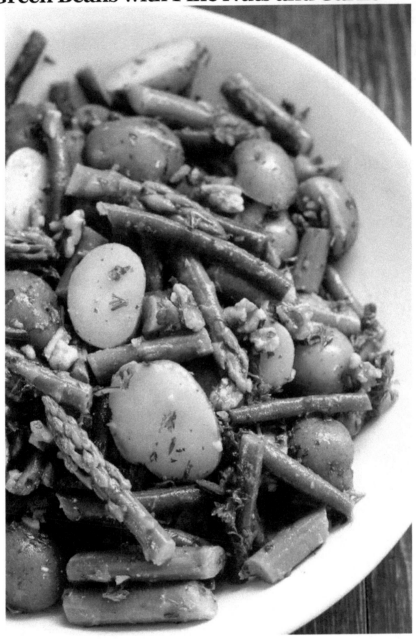

Difficulty Level: 2/5

Preparation time: *10 minutes*

Cooking time: *20 minutes*

Servings: *4-6*

Ingredients:

1 pound green beans, trimmed

1 head garlic (10 to 12 cloves), smashed

2 tablespoons extra-virgin olive oil

½ teaspoon kosher salt

¼ teaspoon red pepper flakes

1 tablespoon white wine vinegar

¼ cup pine nuts, toasted

Directions:

 Preheat the oven to 425°F. Line a baking sheet with parchment paper or foil.

 In a large bowl, combine the green beans, garlic, olive oil, salt, and red pepper flakes and mix together. Arrange in a single layer on the baking sheet. Roast for 10 minutes, stir, and roast for another 10 minutes, or until golden brown.

 Mix the cooked green beans with the vinegar and top with the pine nuts.

COOKING TIP: To cut down on prep time, purchase pre-trimmed green beans. They are typically sold in 1-pound bags in the vegetable area at your local grocery store.

Nutrition:

Calories: 165

Total fat: 13g

Saturated fat: 1g

Cholesterol: 0mg

Sodium: 150mg

Potassium: 325mg

Total Carbohydrates: 12g

Fiber: 4g

Sugars: 4g

Protein: 4g

Magnesium: 52mg

Calcium: 60mg

Cucumbers with Feta, Mint, and Sumac

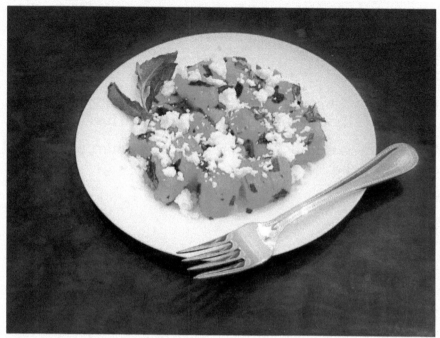

Difficulty Level: 1/5

Preparation time: *15 minutes*

Cooking time: *0 minutes*

Servings: *4*

Ingredients:

1 tablespoon extra-virgin olive oil

1 tablespoon lemon juice

2 teaspoons ground sumac

½ teaspoon kosher salt

2 hothouse or English cucumbers, diced

¼ cup crumbled feta cheese

1 tablespoon fresh mint, chopped

1 tablespoon fresh parsley, chopped

⅛ teaspoon red pepper flakes

Directions:

In a large bowl, whisk together the olive oil, lemon juice, sumac, and salt. Add the cucumber and feta cheese and toss well.

Transfer to a serving dish and sprinkle with the mint, parsley, and red pepper flakes.

Nutrition:

Calories: 85

Total fat: 6g

Saturated fat: 2g

Cholesterol: 8mg

Sodium: 230mg

Potassium: 295mg

Total Carbohydrates: 8g

Fiber: 1g

Sugars: 3g

Protein: 4g

Magnesium: 27mg

Calcium: 80mg

Cherry Tomato Bruschetta
Difficulty Level: 1/5

Preparation time: *15 minutes*

Cooking time: *0 minutes*

Servings: *4*

Ingredients:

8 ounces assorted cherry tomatoes, halved

⅓ cup fresh herbs, chopped (such as basil, parsley, tarragon, dill)

1 tablespoon extra-virgin olive oil

¼ teaspoon kosher salt

⅛ teaspoon freshly ground black pepper

¼ cup ricotta cheese

4 slices whole-wheat bread, toasted

Directions:

Combine the tomatoes, herbs, olive oil, salt, and black pepper in a medium bowl and mix gently.

Spread 1 tablespoon of ricotta cheese onto each slice of toast. Spoon one-quarter of the tomato mixture onto each bruschetta. If desired, garnish with more herbs.

Nutrition:

Calories: 100

Total fat: 6g

Saturated fat: 1g

Cholesterol: 5mg

Sodium: 135mg

Potassium: 210mg

Total Carbohydrates: 10g

Fiber: 2g

Sugars: 2g

Protein: 4g

Magnesium: 22mg

Calcium: 60mg

Roasted Red Pepper Hummus
Difficulty Level: 1/5

Preparation time: *15 minutes*

Cooking time: *0 minutes*

Servings: *2 cups*

Ingredients:

1 (15-ounce) can low-sodium chickpeas, drained and rinsed

3 ounces jarred roasted red bell peppers, drained

3 tablespoons tahini

3 tablespoons lemon juice

1 garlic clove, peeled

¾ teaspoon kosher salt

¼ teaspoon freshly ground black pepper

3 tablespoons extra-virgin olive oil

¼ teaspoon cayenne pepper (optional)

Fresh herbs, chopped, for garnish (optional)

Directions:

In a food processor, add the chickpeas, red bell peppers, tahini, lemon juice, garlic, salt, and black pepper. Pulse 5 to 7 times. Add the olive oil and process until smooth. Add the cayenne pepper and garnish with chopped herbs, if desired.

Nutrition:

Per serving (1/4 cup)

Calories: 130

Total fat: 8g

Saturated fat: 1g

Cholesterol: 0mg

Sodium: 150mg

Potassium: 125mg

Total Carbohydrates: 11g

Fiber: 2g

Sugars: 1g

Protein: 4g

Magnesium: 20mg

Calcium: 48mg

Roasted Rosemary Olives
Difficulty Level: 2/5

Preparation time: *5 minutes*

Cooking time: *25 minutes*

Servings: *4*

Ingredients:

1 cup mixed variety olives, pitted and rinsed

2 tablespoons lemon juice

1 tablespoon extra-virgin olive oil

6 garlic cloves, peeled

4 rosemary sprigs

Directions:

Preheat the oven to 400°F. Line the baking sheet with parchment paper or foil.

Combine the olives, lemon juice, olive oil, and garlic in a medium bowl and mix together. Spread in a single layer on the prepared baking sheet. Sprinkle on the rosemary. Roast for 25 minutes, tossing halfway through.

Remove the rosemary leaves from the stem and place in a serving bowl. Add the olives and mix before serving.

Nutrition:

Per serving

Calories: 100

Total fat: 9g

Saturated fat: 1g

Cholesterol: 0mg

Sodium: 260mg

Potassium: 31mg

Total Carbohydrates: 4g

Fiber: 0g

Sugars: 0g

Protein: 0g

Magnesium: 3mg

Calcium: 11mg

Spiced Maple Nuts
Difficulty Level: 2/5

Preparation time: *5 minutes*

Cooking time: *10 minutes*

Servings: *2 cups*

Ingredients:

2 cups raw walnuts or pecans (or a mix of nuts)

1 teaspoon extra-virgin olive oil

1 teaspoon ground sumac

½ teaspoon pure maple syrup

¼ teaspoon kosher salt

¼ teaspoon ground ginger

2 to 4 rosemary sprigs

Directions:

Preheat the oven to 350°F. Line a baking sheet with parchment paper or foil.

In a large bowl, combine the nuts, olive oil, sumac, maple syrup, salt, and ginger; mix together. Spread in a single layer on the prepared baking sheet. Add the rosemary. Roast for 8 to 10 minutes, or until golden and fragrant.

Remove the rosemary leaves from the stems and place in a serving bowl. Add the nuts and toss to combine before serving.

Nutrition:

Per serving (1/4 cup)

Calories: 175

Total fat: 18g

Saturated fat: 2g

Cholesterol: 0mg

Sodium: 35mg

Potassium: 110mg

Total Carbohydrates: 4g

Fiber: 2g

Sugars: 1g

Protein: 3g

Magnesium: 35mg

Calcium: 23mg

Greek Turkey Burger

Difficulty Level: 2/5

Preparation time: 10 *minutes*

Cooking time: *10 minutes*

Servings: *4*

Ingredients:

1 pound ground turkey

1 medium zucchini, grated

¼ cup whole-wheat bread crumbs

¼ cup red onion, minced

¼ cup crumbled feta cheese

1 large egg, beaten

1 garlic clove, minced

1 tablespoon fresh oregano, chopped

1 teaspoon kosher salt

¼ teaspoon freshly ground black pepper

1 tablespoon extra-virgin olive oil

Directions:

In a large bowl, combine the turkey, zucchini, bread crumbs, onion, feta cheese, egg, garlic, oregano, salt, and black pepper, and mix well. Shape into 4 equal patties.

Heat the olive oil in a large nonstick grill pan or skillet over medium-high heat. Add the burgers to the pan and reduce the heat to medium. Cook on one side for 5 minutes, then flip and cook the other side for 5 minutes more.

SUBSTITUTION TIP: Any summer squash can be used in this recipe, so feel free to swap out the zucchini for yellow squash or pattypan squash.

Nutrition:

Per serving

Calories: 285

Total fat: 16g

Saturated fat: 5g

Cholesterol: 139mg

Sodium: 465mg

Potassium: 415mg

Total Carbohydrates: 9g

Fiber: 2g

Sugars: 2g

Protein: 26g

Magnesium: 40mg

Calcium: 90mg

Za'atar Chicken Tenders
Difficulty Level: 2/5

Preparation time: *5 minutes*

Cooking time: *15 minutes*

Servings: *4*

Ingredients:

Olive oil cooking spray

1 pound chicken tenders

1½ tablespoons za'atar

½ teaspoon kosher salt

¼ teaspoon freshly ground black pepper

Directions:

Preheat the oven to 450°F. Line a baking sheet with parchment paper or foil and lightly spray with olive oil cooking spray.

In a large bowl, combine the chicken, za'atar, salt, and black pepper. Mix together well, covering the chicken tenders fully. Arrange in a single layer on the baking sheet and bake for 15 minutes, turning the chicken over once halfway through the cooking time.

Nutrition:

Per serving

Calories: 145

Total fat: 4g

Saturated fat: 1g

Cholesterol: 83mg

Sodium: 190mg

Potassium: 390mg

Total Carbohydrates: 0g

Fiber: 0g

Sugars: 0g

Protein: 26g

Magnesium: 37mg

Calcium: 13mg

Yogurt-Marinated Chicken Kebabs

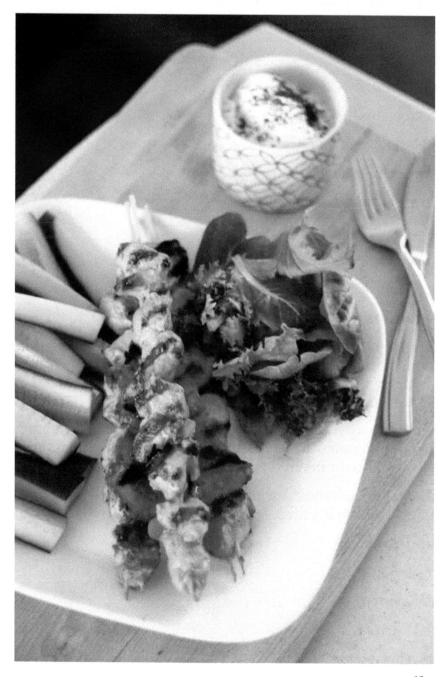

Difficulty Level: 2/5

Preparation time: 10 *minutes*

Cooking time: *20 minutes*

Servings: *4*

Ingredients:

½ cup plain Greek yogurt

1 tablespoon lemon juice

½ teaspoon ground cumin

½ teaspoon ground coriander

½ teaspoon kosher salt

¼ teaspoon cayenne pepper

1½ pound skinless, boneless chicken breast, cut into 1-inch cubes

Directions:

In a large bowl or zip-top bag, combine the yogurt, lemon juice, cumin, coriander, salt, and cayenne pepper. Mix together thoroughly and then add the chicken. Marinate for at least 30 minutes, and up to overnight in the refrigerator.

Preheat the oven to 425°F. Line a baking sheet with parchment paper or foil. Remove the chicken from the marinade and thread it on 4 bamboo or metal skewers.

Bake for 20 minutes, turning the chicken over once halfway through the cooking time.

Nutrition:

Per serving

Calories: 170

Total fat: 4g

Saturated fat: 1g

Cholesterol: 92mg

Sodium: 390mg

Potassium: 515mg

Total Carbohydrates: 1g

Fiber: 0g

Sugars: 1g

Protein: 31g

Magnesium: 40mg

Calcium: 35mg

Honey Ricotta with Espresso and Chocolate Chips

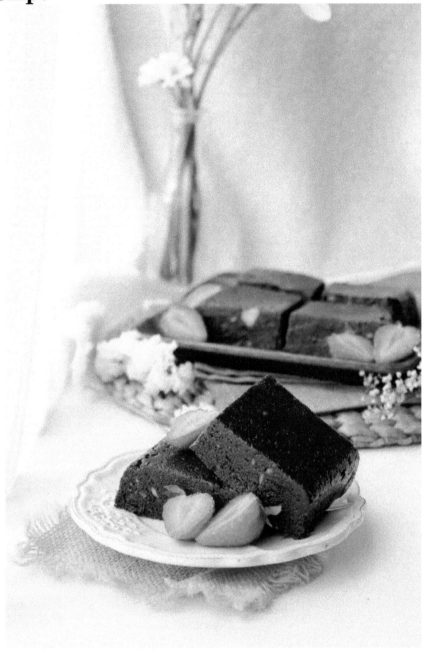

Difficulty Level: 1/5

Preparation time: *5 minutes*

Cooking time: *0 minutes*

Servings: *2*

Ingredients:

8 ounces ricotta cheese

2 tablespoons honey

2 tablespoons espresso, chilled or room temperature

1 teaspoon dark chocolate chips or chocolate shavings

Directions:

In a medium bowl, whip together the ricotta cheese and honey until light and smooth, 4 to 5 minutes.

Spoon the ricotta cheese–honey mixture evenly into 2 dessert bowls. Drizzle 1 tablespoon espresso into each dish and sprinkle with chocolate chips or shavings.

SUBSTITUTION TIP: Regular or decaf black coffee can be used in place of the espresso.

Nutrition:

Per serving

Calories: 235

Total fat: 10g

Saturated fat: 6g

Cholesterol: 35mg

Sodium: 115mg

Potassium: 170mg

Total Carbohydrates: 25g

Fiber: 0g

Sugars: 19g

Protein: 13g

Magnesium: 30mg

Calcium: 310mg

Figs with Mascarpone and Honey

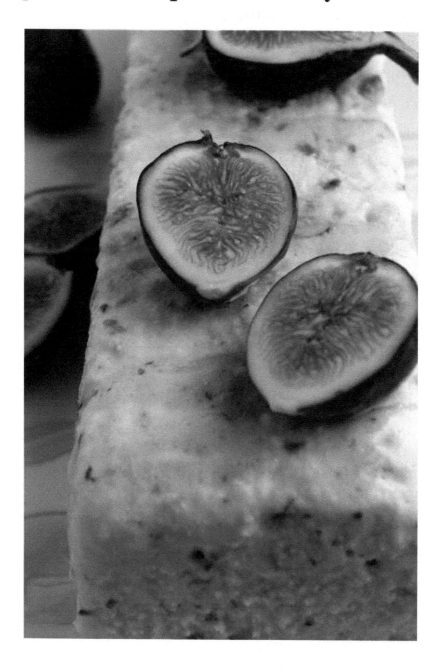

Difficulty Level: 2/5

Preparation time: 5 minutes

Cooking time: 5 minutes

Servings: 4

Ingredients:

⅓ cup walnuts, chopped

8 fresh figs, halved

¼ cup mascarpone cheese

1 tablespoon honey

¼ teaspoon flaked sea salt

Directions:

In a skillet over medium heat, toast the walnuts, stirring often, 3 to 5 minutes.

Arrange the figs cut-side up on a plate or platter. Using your finger, make a small depression in the cut side of each fig and fill with mascarpone cheese. Sprinkle with a bit of the walnuts, drizzle with the honey, and add a tiny pinch of sea salt.

Nutrition:

Per serving

Calories: 200

Total fat: 13g

Saturated fat: 4g

Cholesterol: 18mg

Sodium: 105mg

Potassium: 230mg

Total Carbohydrates: 24g

Fiber: 3g

Sugars: 18g

Protein: 3g

Magnesium: 30mg

Calcium: 53mg

Pistachio-Stuffed Dates

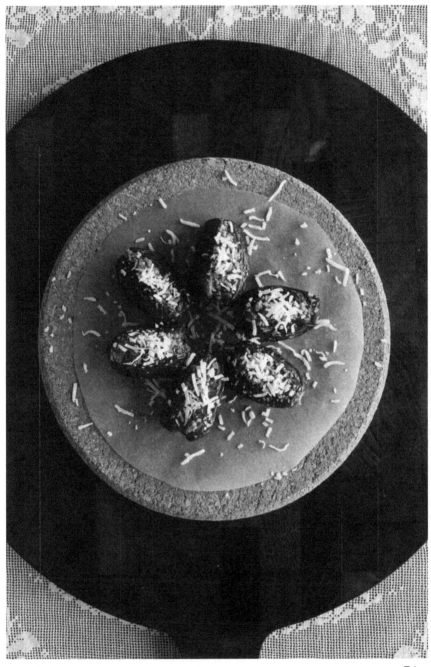

Difficulty Level: 1/5

Preparation time: 10 *minutes*

Cooking time: *0 minutes*

Servings: *4*

Ingredients:

½ cup unsalted pistachios, shelled

¼ teaspoon kosher salt

8 Medjool dates, pitted

Directions:

In a food processor, add the pistachios and salt. Process until combined to a chunky nut butter, 3 to 5 minutes.

Split open the dates and spoon the pistachio nut butter into each half.

Nutrition:

Per serving

Calories: 220

Total fat: 7g

Saturated fat: 1g

Cholesterol: 0mg

Sodium: 70mg

Potassium: 490mg

Total Carbohydrates: 41g

Fiber: 5g

Sugars: 33g

Protein: 4g

Magnesium: 43mg

Calcium: 47mg

Yogurt Tahini Dressing

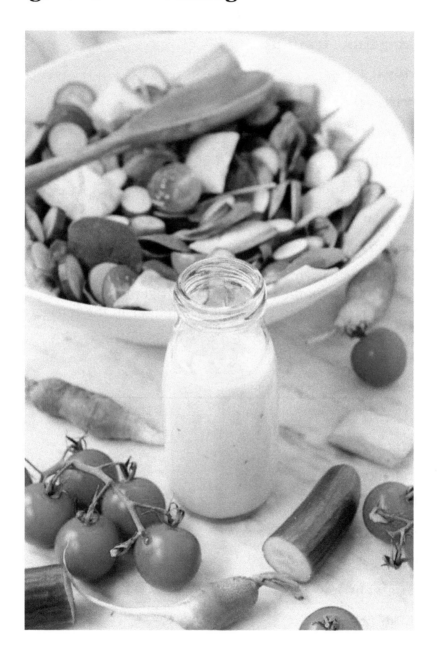

Difficulty Level: 1/5

Preparation time: 5 *minutes*

Cooking time: *0 minutes*

Servings: *1 cup*

Ingredients:

½ cup plain Greek yogurt

⅓ cup tahini

¼ cup freshly squeezed orange juice

½ teaspoon kosher salt

Directions:

In a medium bowl, whisk together the yogurt, tahini, orange juice, and salt until smooth. Place in the refrigerator until ready to serve. Store leftovers in an airtight container in the refrigerator for up to 5 days.

Nutrition:

Per serving (2 tablespoons)

Calories: 70

Total fat: 2g

Saturated fat: 1g

Cholesterol: 0mg

Sodium: 80mg

Potassium: 85mg

Total Carbohydrates: 4g

Fiber: 1g

Sugars: 1g

Protein: 4g

Magnesium: 12mg

Calcium: 66mg

Portable Packed Picnic Pieces

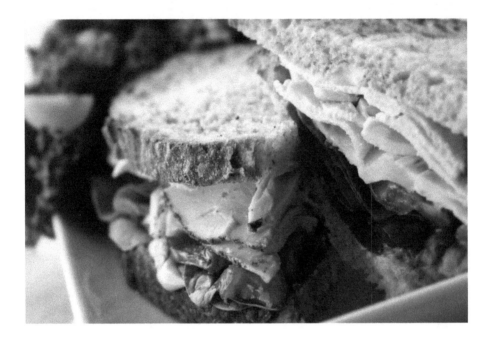

Difficulty Level: 1/5

Preparation time: 10 minutes

Cooking time: 0 minutes

Servings: 1

Ingredients:

1-slice of whole-wheat bread, cut into bite-size pieces

10-pcs cherry tomatoes

¼-oz. aged cheese, sliced

6-pcs oil-cured olives

Directions:

Pack each of the ingredients in a portable container to serve you while snacking on the go.

Nutrition:

Calories: 197

Total Fats: 9g

Fiber: 4g

Carbohydrates: 22g

Protein: 7g

Naturally Nutty & Buttery Banana Bowl

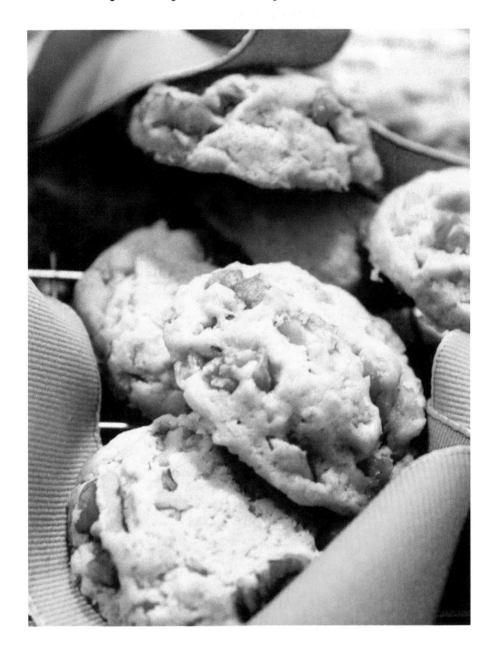

Difficulty Level: 1/5

Preparation time: minutes

Cooking time: 0 minutes

Servings: 4

Ingredients:

4-cups vanilla Greek yogurt

2-pcs medium-sized bananas, sliced

¼-cup creamy and natural peanut butter

1-tsp ground nutmeg

¼-cup flaxseed meal

Directions:

Divide the yogurt equally between four serving bowls. Top each yogurt bowl with the banana slices.

Place the peanut butter in a microwave-safe bowl. Melt the peanut butter in your microwave for 40 seconds. Drizzle one tablespoon of the melted peanut butter over the bananas for each bowl.

To serve, sprinkle over with the ground nutmeg and flax-seed meal.

Nutrition:

Calories: 370

Total Fats: 10.6g

Fiber: 4.7g

Carbohydrates: 47.7g

Protein: 22.7g

Cannellini Beans with Rosemary and Garlic Aioli

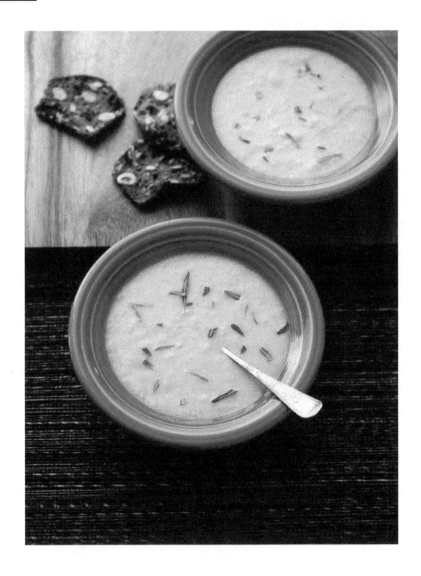

Difficulty Level: 2/5

Preparation time: 10 minutes

Cooking time: 10 minutes

Servings: 4

Ingredients:

4 cups cooked cannellini beans (see tip)

4 cups water

½ teaspoon salt

3 tablespoons olive oil

2 tablespoons chopped fresh rosemary

½ cup Garlic Aioli

¼ teaspoon freshly ground black pepper

Directions:

In a medium saucepan over medium heat, combine the cannellini beans, water, and salt. Bring to a boil. Cook for 5 minutes. Drain.

In a skillet over medium heat, heat the olive oil.

Add the beans. Stir in the rosemary and aioli. Reduce the heat to medium-low and cook, stirring, just to heat through. Season with pepper and serve.

Nutrition:

Calories: 545

Total Fats: 36g

Saturated Fat: 6g

Fiber: 14g

Carbohydrates: 42g

Protein: 15g

Sodium: 448mg

Ful Medames

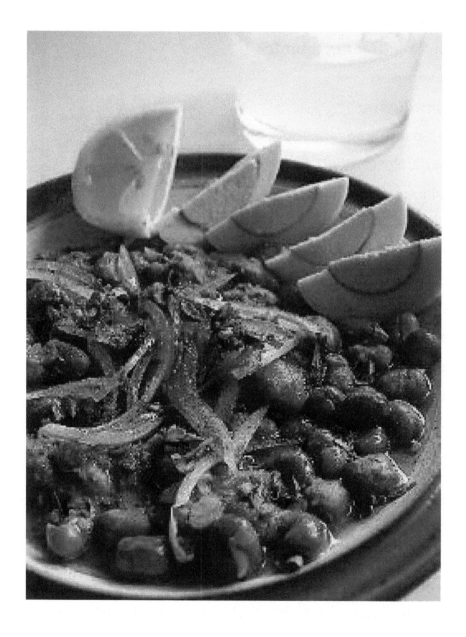

Difficulty Level: 2/5

Preparation time: 15 minutes

Cooking time: 15 minutes

Servings: 6

Ingredients:

1 (15-ounce) can fava beans, undrained

4 garlic cloves, minced

1 tablespoon ground cumin

⅛ teaspoon salt

⅛ teaspoon freshly ground black pepper

½ cup freshly squeezed lemon juice

¼ cup olive oil

1 sweet onion, chopped, divided

2 ripe tomatoes, diced, divided

2 cups finely chopped fresh parsley, divided

Directions:

In a medium saucepan over medium heat, combine the fava beans with their liquid, garlic, cumin, salt, and pepper. Bring to a boil.

Using a potato masher or fork, partially mash the fava beans. Continue to cook over medium heat for 10 minutes more.

Stir in the lemon juice, olive oil, and half each of the onion, tomatoes, and parsley. Taste and season with more salt and pepper, as needed. Remove from the heat.

Spoon the bean mixture into a serving dish and top while hot with the remaining onion, tomatoes, and parsley.

Nutrition:

Calories: 183

Total Fats: 9g

Saturated Fat: 2g

Fiber: 6g

Carbohydrates: 20g

Protein: 15g

Sodium: 74mg

Fresh Sauce Pasta

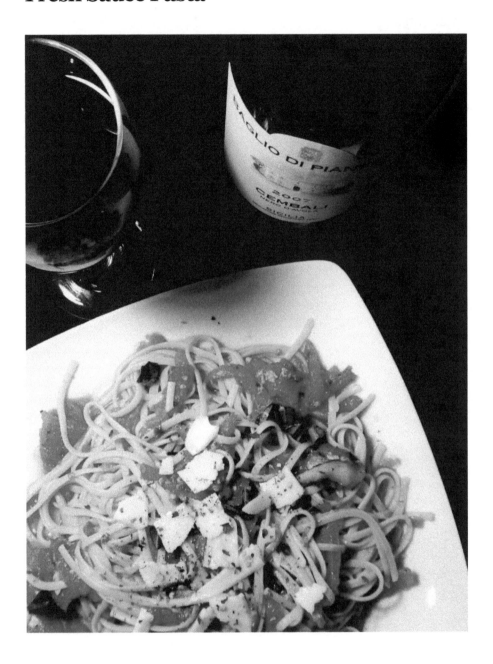

Difficulty Level: 2/5

Preparation time: 15 minutes

Cooking time: 15 minutes

Servings: 4

Ingredients:

⅛ teaspoon salt, plus more for cooking the pasta

1 pound penne pasta

¼ cup olive oil

1 garlic clove, crushed

3 cups chopped scallions, white and green parts

3 tomatoes, diced

2 tablespoons chopped fresh basil

⅛ teaspoon freshly ground black pepper

Freshly grated Parmesan cheese, for serving

Directions:

Bring a large pot of salted water to a boil over high heat. Drop in the pasta, stir, and return the water to a boil. Boil the pasta for about 6 minutes or until al dente.

A couple minutes before the pasta is completely cooked, in a medium saucepan over medium heat, heat the olive oil.

Add the garlic and cook for 30 seconds.

Stir in the scallions and tomatoes. Cover the pan and cook for 2 to 3 minutes.

Drain the pasta and add it to the vegetables. Stir in the basil and season with the salt and pepper. Top with the Parmesan cheese.

Nutrition:

Calories: 477

Total Fats: 16g

Saturated Fat: 2g

Fiber: 3g

Carbohydrates: 72g

Protein: 15g

Sodium: 120mg

Penne in Tomato and Caper Sauce

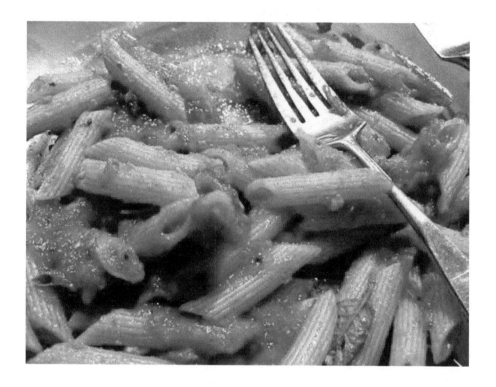

Difficulty Level: 2/5

Preparation time: 10 minutes

Cooking time: 15 minutes

Servings: 4

Ingredients:

2 tablespoons olive oil

2 garlic cloves, minced

1 cup sliced cherry tomatoes

2 cups Basic Tomato Basil Sauce, or store-bought

1 cup capers, drained and rinsed

Salt

4 cups penne pasta

Directions:

Set a large pot of salted water over high heat to boil.

In a medium saucepan over medium heat, heat the olive oil. Add the garlic and cook for 30 seconds. Add the cherry tomatoes and cook for 2 to 3 minutes.

Pour in the tomato sauce and bring the mixture to a boil. Stir in the capers and turn off the heat.

Once boiling add the pasta to the pot of water and cook for about 7 minutes until al dente.

Drain the pasta and stir it into the sauce. Toss gently and cook over medium heat for 1 minute or until warmed through.

Nutrition:

Calories: 329

Total Fats: 8g

Saturated Fat: 1g

Fiber: 6g

Carbohydrates: 55g

Protein: 10g

Sodium: 612mg

Tahini Sauce

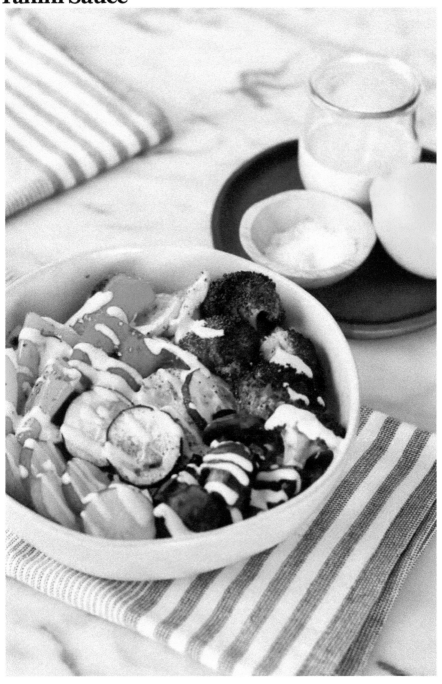

Difficulty Level: 1/5

Preparation time: 15 minutes

Cooking time: 0 minutes

Servings: 2 cups

Ingredients:

3 garlic cloves, minced or mashed into a paste

½ cup tahini

½ cup freshly squeezed lemon juice

1 cup water

¼ teaspoon ground cumin

⅛ teaspoon salt

4 cups penne pasta

Directions:

In a small bowl, whisk the garlic, tahini, lemon juice, water, cumin, and salt until it develops into a smooth paste. Refrigerate in an airtight container for up to 1 month.

Nutrition:

Per serving (1tablespoon)

Calories: 47

Total Fats: 4g

Saturated Fat: 1g

Fiber: 1g

Carbohydrates: 2g

Protein: 1g

Sodium: 30mg

Basil Pesto

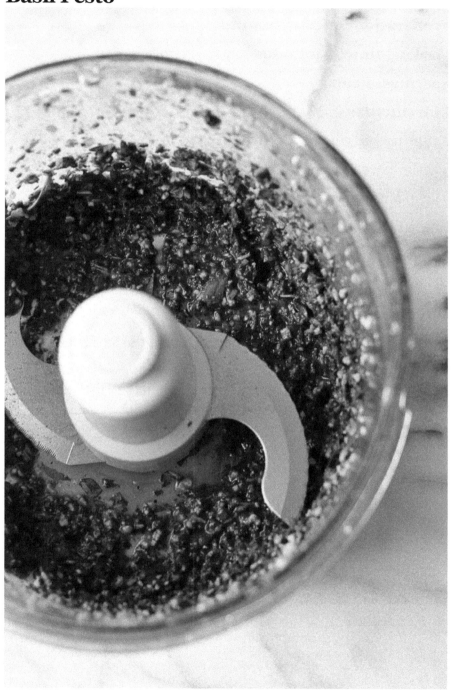

Difficulty Level: 2/5

Preparation time: 15 minutes

Cooking time: 0 minutes

Servings: 1 cup

Ingredients:

2 cups packed chopped fresh basil

3 garlic cloves, peeled

¼ cup pine nuts

½ cup olive oil

½ teaspoon salt

½ cup freshly grated Parmesan cheese

Directions:

1.   In a food processor or blender, combine the basil, garlic, and pine nuts. Pulse until coarsely chopped.

Add the olive oil, salt, and Parmesan cheese. Process for 5 minutes until you have a smooth paste.

Refrigerate in an airtight container for up to 3 weeks, or freeze for up to 1 month

Nutrition:

Per serving (1tablespoon)

Calories: 81

Total Fats: 9g

Saturated Fat: 2g

Fiber: 0g

Carbohydrates: 1g

Protein: 2g

Sodium: 91mg

Barley Porridge

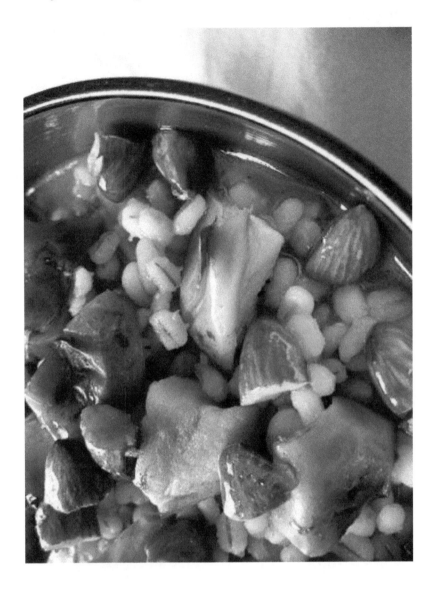

Difficulty Level: 2/5

Preparation time: 25 minutes

Cooking time: 5 minutes

Servings: 4

Ingredients:

1 cup barley

1 cup wheat berries

2 cups unsweetened almond milk, plus more for serving

2 cups water

½ cup blueberries

½ cup pomegranate seeds

½ cup hazelnuts, toasted and chopped

¼ cup honey

Directions:

In a medium saucepan over medium-high heat, place the barley, wheat berries, almond milk, and water. Bring to a boil, reduce the heat to low, and simmer for about 25 minutes, stirring frequently until the grains are very tender.

Top each serving with almond milk, 2 tablespoons of blueberries, 2 tablespoons of pomegranate seeds, 2 tablespoons of hazelnuts, and 1 tablespoon of honey.

Nutrition:

Calories: 354;

Total Fat: 8g;

Saturated Fat: 1g;

Carbohydrates: 63g;

Fiber: 10g;

Protein: 11g

Spiced Almond Pancakes

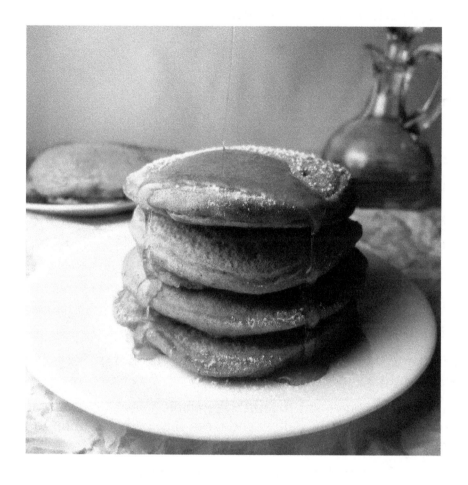

Difficulty Level: 2/5

Preparation time: 10 minutes

Cooking time: 20 minutes

Servings: 6

Ingredients:

1 pound chicken breasts, cut into medium chunks

12 ounces zucchini, sliced

2 tablespoons olive oil

2 garlic cloves, minced

2 tablespoons parmesan, grated

1 tablespoon parsley, chopped

Salt and black pepper to taste

Directions:

In a large bowl, whisk the almond milk, coconut oil, eggs, and honey until blended.

In a medium bowl, sift together the whole-wheat flour, almond flour, baking powder, baking soda, sea salt, and cinnamon until well mixed.

Add the flour mixture to the milk mixture and whisk until just combined.

Grease a large skillet with coconut oil and place it over medium-high heat.

Add the pancake batter in ½-cup measures, about 3 for a large skillet. Cook for about 3 minutes until the edges are firm, the bottom is golden, and the bubbles on the surface break. Flip and cook for about 2 minutes more until the other side is golden brown and the pancakes are cooked through. Transfer to a plate and wipe the skillet with a clean paper towel.

Re-grease the skillet and repeat until the remaining batter is used.
Serve the pancakes warm with fresh fruit, if desired.

Nutrition:

Calories: 286;

Total Fat: 17g;

Saturated Fat: 12g;

Carbohydrates: 27g;

Fiber: 1g;

Protein: 6g

Artichoke Frittata

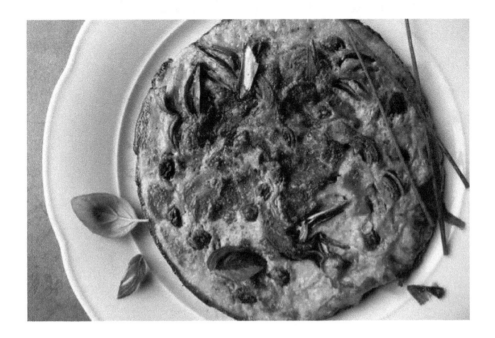

Difficulty Level: 2/5

Preparation time: 10 minutes

Cooking time: 15 minutes

Servings: 4

Ingredients:

8 large eggs

¼ cup grated Asiago cheese

1 tablespoon chopped fresh basil

1 teaspoon chopped fresh oregano

Pinch sea salt

Pinch freshly ground black pepper

1 teaspoon extra-virgin olive oil

1 teaspoon minced garlic

1 cup canned, water-packed, quartered artichoke hearts, drained

1 tomato, chopped

Directions:

Preheat the oven to broil.

In a medium bowl, whisk the eggs, Asiago cheese, basil, oregano, sea salt, and pepper to blend.

Place a large ovenproof skillet over medium-high heat and add the olive oil. Add the garlic and sauté for 1 minute.

Remove the skillet from the heat and pour in the egg mixture.

Return the skillet to the heat and evenly sprinkle the artichoke hearts and tomato over the eggs.

Cook the frittata without stirring for about 8 minutes, or until the center is set.

Place the skillet under the broiler for about 1 minute, or until the top is lightly browned and puffed.

Cut the frittata into 4 pieces and serve.

Nutrition:

Calories: 199;

Total Fat: 13g;

Saturated Fat: 5g;

Carbohydrates: 5g;

Fiber: 2g;

Protein: 16g

Parmesan Mashed Potatoes with Olive Oil, Garlic, & Parsley
Difficulty Level: 2/5

Preparation time: 5 minutes

Cooking time: 30 minutes

Servings: 4

Ingredients:

5 pounds red skinned potatoes (chopped into 2 inch pieces)

2 heads roasted garlic

4 tablespoons garlic powder

3 cups heavy cream

1/2 pound Parmesan cheese

1/4 cup fresh parsley (chopped)

1/4 cup olive oil (Pompeian, I love the Mediterranean blend!)

pepper

salt

olive oil (additional, to drizzle & fresh chopped parsley to garnish, optional)

Directions:

Boil the potatoes in enough water to cover until fork tender. Drain. Place the potatoes back into the pot on medium, and mash best you can with a potato masher to release the steam. Pour in the heavy cream, & finish mashing the potatoes. Stir the mixture to combine. Stir in the Parmesan cheese, garlic, & fresh chopped parsley. Drizzle in the olive oil, a little at a time - stirring after each drizzle, until all the olive oil is combined. Season with salt & pepper to taste.

Scoop into your serving vessel; drizzle with olive oil and sprinkle on chopped parsley to garnish if desired

Nutrition: (Per serving)

1570 Calories;

0.113g fat;

0.109g carbs;

0.38g protein;

Greek Cauliflower Rice with Feta and Olives
Difficulty Level: 2/5

Preparation time: 5 minutes

Cooking time: 30 minutes

Servings: 4

Ingredients:

1 shallot (large, diced)

1 tablespoon coconut oil

1 pound cauliflower (aged or shredded in food processor, you can buy it pre-shredded at Trader Joe's in the products section)

1 cup of crumbled feta cheese

1/2 cup sliced black olives (kalamata is great, but every black olive does with it)

1/3 cup parsley (finely chopped, plus more for garnish)

salt

pepper

Directions:

Heat coconut oil in a frying pan over medium heat. When the oil sparkles, add the diced shallot. Sauté until transparent.

Put the cauliflower rice in the pan. Cook for 10-15 minutes, stirring occasionally. Brown the cauliflower a little and then remove from the heat. Stir in the parsley, olives and feta and season with salt and pepper. Garnish with extra parsley if desired. Serve hot.

Nutrition: (Per serving)

200 Calories;

0.13g fat;

0.15g carbs;

0.9g protein

Lightning Source UK Ltd.
Milton Keynes UK
UKHW020656310521
384668UK00001B/107